Navigating Rheumatoid Arthritis

A Comprehensive Handbook for Empowered Living, Wellness, and Proactive Health Management

By Dr. Edna Walton

Copyright © 2023 by Edna Walton

All rights reserved. No part of this publication may be reproduced, distributed, or transmitted in any form or by any means, including photocopying, recording, or other electronic or mechanical methods, without the prior written permission of the publisher, except in the case of brief quotations embodied in critical reviews and certain other noncommercial uses permitted by copyright law.

About the Author

Edna Walton is a passionate advocate for health and well-being, focusing on empowering individuals navigating the challenges of Rheumatoid Arthritis (RA). As a seasoned rheumatologist, Edna brings a wealth of professional expertise and a deep understanding of the physical and emotional impact of RA.

Her commitment to patient-centric care goes beyond the clinic, as evidenced by her dedication to providing accessible and comprehensive information. Through her writing, Edna aims to demystify the complexities of RA, offering guidance and support to those on their journey to manage and thrive despite the condition.

Edna Walton's holistic approach combines medical insights with a compassionate understanding of the human experience, bridging clinical knowledge and the daily realities faced by individuals living with RA. Her work seeks to inspire hope, foster resilience, and encourage a proactive approach to achieving a fulfilling life with Rheumatoid Arthritis.

Beyond her medical practice, Edna is an avid advocate for patient education, regularly contributing to health forums and community outreach programs. Her commitment to raising awareness about RA extends to the written word, where she shares her expertise to empower readers confidently with the tools they need to navigate the challenges of RA.

In "Navigating Rheumatoid Arthritis," Edna Walton invites readers to embark on a journey of understanding, resilience, and empowerment. Her unique blend of medical knowledge and empathetic communication serves as a guide for individuals seeking not just to manage RA but to live a vibrant and fulfilling life despite its challenges.

Table of contents

Introduction

Welcome to the pages of "Navigating Rheumatoid Arthritis: A Comprehensive Handbook for Empowered Living, Wellness, and Proactive Health Management." As a dedicated rheumatologist, I extend a heartfelt invitation to embark on a transformative journey through the intricate landscape of Rheumatoid Arthritis (RA). These words are more than ink on paper; they represent the culmination of experiences, empathy, and a profound desire to empower those who navigate the challenges of RA.

Having witnessed the trials and triumphs of individuals grappling with RA, this book is a testament to the resilience and courage that permeate the lives of those touched by this condition. It draws inspiration from the untold stories within my practice – stories of strength, perseverance, and the unwavering spirit of individuals confronting the complexities of RA daily.

In crafting this guide, I intend to extend beyond the traditional realm of clinical advice. It is an endeavor to offer more than medical insights; it's a companion, a source of understanding, and a guide that aspires to empower you with the knowledge and tools needed to navigate the often challenging path of Rheumatoid Arthritis.

The essence of this book lies in the belief that knowledge is empowerment. Each chapter is a step towards demystifying RA, delving into its physical, emotional, and practical dimensions. I hope that, armed with this understanding, you will not only manage the condition more effectively but also find the strength to live a life not defined by RA but one that transcends it.

Through these pages, I share clinical expertise and a personal connection to the struggles and victories entwined with RA. This book bridges the medical world and the deeply personal experiences of those living with RA. It is an expression of empathy, a nod to the challenges you face, and an acknowledgment of the strength that resides within you.

As we embark on this journey together, envision these words as information and a source of empowerment. May "Navigating Rheumatoid Arthritis" be a guiding light, providing insights, strategies, and a sense of companionship as you navigate the unique landscape of RA.

Chapter One: Understanding Rheumatoid Arthritis

In this chapter, we embark on a comprehensive exploration of Rheumatoid Arthritis (RA). We unravel the intricate nature of RA, distinguishing it from other forms of arthritis providing a clear explanation of this autoimmune condition. Moving forward, we delve into the multifaceted contributors to RA development, exploring common risk factors and their implications.

Within the realm of symptoms, we meticulously examine the nuanced aspects of RA, underscoring the critical importance of early detection and prompt medical attention. Lastly, we explore the profound effects of RA on daily life, acknowledging both the physical and emotional dimensions of this intricate journey.

Definition and Overview of RA

Rheumatoid Arthritis (RA) stands as a chronic autoimmune disorder that primarily targets the joints, triggering persistent inflammation, pain, and potential joint damage. Unlike osteoarthritis, which commonly arises from mechanical wear and tear on joints, RA's origin lies in the body's immune system mistakenly attacking healthy joint tissues.

At the core of RA lies the inflammation of the synovium, a protective membrane surrounding the joints. Over time, this inflammation can lead to the erosion of cartilage, bone, and even nearby ligaments, resulting in joint deformities, mobility issues, and chronic pain. RA tends to affect multiple joints, commonly impacting the hands, wrists, feet, elbows, and knees. Its hallmark characteristic often involves symmetrical joint involvement, where joints on both sides of the body are affected.

Distinguishing RA from other forms of arthritis, especially osteoarthritis, is pivotal for accurate diagnosis and targeted treatment. While osteoarthritis typically affects specific joints due to wear and tear, RA manifests as a systemic disease, impacting not only the joints but also potentially affecting various organs and bodily systems. Unlike osteoarthritis, RA can lead to general symptoms such as fatigue, fever, and weight loss, indicative of its systemic nature.

A comprehensive understanding of these distinctions is essential for healthcare providers to initiate timely interventions and personalized treatment plans. Early diagnosis becomes pivotal in RA management, as it allows for the implementation of therapies aimed at controlling inflammation, preserving joint function, and enhancing the overall quality of life for individuals affected by this complex condition.

Causes and Risk Factors

The genesis of Rheumatoid Arthritis (RA) is a multifaceted journey, intricately woven by genetic predisposition, environmental influences, and immunological intricacies. The exploration of these contributing factors reveals a complex interplay. Genetic susceptibility, particularly associated with specific HLA (human leukocyte antigen) genes, predisposes individuals to RA. Environmental triggers, ranging from infections to exposure to specific pollutants, can act as catalysts, initiating or amplifying the autoimmune response that characterizes RA.

The immune system emerges as a central player in RA development. An aberrant immune response sets the stage, activating T and B cells. These immune cells release inflammatory mediators, perpetuating chronic inflammation. The synovium, the membranous lining encapsulating the joints, becomes a focal point of this immune assault, resulting in sustained inflammation and eventual joint damage.

Age and Gender Dynamics: RA typically manifests between the ages of 30 and 60, with women exhibiting a higher susceptibility compared to men. Hormonal influences, particularly those associated with female reproductive cycles, are considered contributory, as evidenced by some women experiencing symptom relief during pregnancy.

Family Ties: A familial backdrop featuring first-degree relatives with RA heightens the risk, underscoring the genetic nuances at play. The hereditary component accentuates the importance of understanding one's familial medical history for proactive health management.

The Smoking Connection: Smoking emerges as a pivotal environmental risk factor for RA. Its impact extends beyond elevating the risk of onset; it also amplifies the severity of the disease. Recognizing and addressing smoking habits becomes integral to comprehensive RA management.

Weighty Matters: Obesity, particularly prevalent in women, is associated with an augmented risk of RA. Adipose tissue is a source of inflammatory substances, contributing to the inflammatory milieu associated with RA. Addressing weight management becomes a crucial facet of holistic RA care.

Infectious Intricacies: Certain infections, such as those instigated by the Epstein-Barr virus or bacteria associated with periodontal disease, have been implicated in elevating the risk of RA. Understanding the infectious underpinnings contributes to a more nuanced approach to RA prevention and management.

This intricate web of causes and risk factors underscores the necessity for a personalized and vigilant healthcare approach. While genetic predispositions and some risk factors may be beyond immediate control, proactive lifestyle adjustments and timely interventions hold the key to navigating the course of RA with resilience and informed decision-making.

Symptoms and Early Detection

Rheumatoid Arthritis (RA) manifests with a rich tapestry of symptoms that, when examined in detail, provide valuable insights into the complexity of this autoimmune disorder. Key symptoms include

Joint Symptoms

Persistent Pain: RA typically presents with persistent joint pain, often described as aching or throbbing. The pain is commonly bilateral, affecting corresponding joints on both sides of the body.

Swelling: Joints affected by RA exhibit swelling due to inflammation of the synovial membrane. This swelling contributes to joint tenderness and warmth.

Morning Stiffness: RA-induced stiffness, particularly in the morning or after periods of inactivity, can last more than an hour. This stiffness is a characteristic feature.

Symmetrical Joint Involvement

RA demonstrates a predilection for symmetrical joint involvement, distinguishing it from other forms of arthritis. Corresponding joints on both sides of the body, such as the wrists, knees, and fingers, are commonly affected.

Specific Joint Affliction

Certain joints are more prone to RA, including the metacarpophalangeal joints of the hands, proximal interphalangeal joints, wrists, and small joints of the feet. The severity can lead to joint deformities and compromised range of motion.

Systemic Symptoms

Fatigue: RA is frequently accompanied by pervasive fatigue unrelated to physical exertion. The profound tiredness can significantly impact daily functioning.

Low-Grade Fever: Systemic inflammation in RA may result in a low-grade fever, contributing to an overall sense of malaise.

Weight Loss: Unintended weight loss is a potential consequence of the systemic impact of RA.

Rheumatoid Nodules

Firm lumps or nodules may sometimes form beneath the skin, typically over pressure points or joints. While not present in all cases, their occurrence is characteristic of advanced RA.

Early detection of RA is a linchpin in the pursuit of optimal outcomes. Recognizing and acting upon initial symptoms are instrumental in curbing the progression of joint damage and systemic consequences. The early phases of RA, often characterized by milder symptoms, necessitate heightened awareness on the part of individuals to promptly seek medical attention when aberrations in joint health or unexplained fatigue arise.

Early diagnosis opens the door to targeted interventions, typically involving disease-modifying antirheumatic drugs (DMARDs) and, in some cases, biologics. These medications not only alleviate symptoms but also exert disease-modifying effects, aiming to slow or halt the destructive course of RA. Moreover, proactive management strategies address the broader impact of RA on daily life, targeting fatigue and enhancing overall well-being.

Impact on Quality of Life

The multifaceted impact of Rheumatoid Arthritis (RA) extends far beyond physical discomfort, permeating various facets of an individual's daily life. The functional constraints RA imposes on joint health manifest in disruptions to routine activities, ranging from the basic functionality of gripping objects to more intricate tasks such as navigating stairs. These limitations can reverberate in the professional sphere, influencing work capacity and productivity, potentially altering career trajectories, and introducing financial uncertainties. Social participation, too, becomes a nuanced endeavor as individuals grapple with the physical toll and discomfort associated with RA, potentially leading to withdrawal from social engagements.

RA's emotional and psychological toll introduces another layer of complexity to its impact on quality of life. Chronic pain and fatigue, intrinsic to RA, create an enduring backdrop of discomfort and exhaustion. The erratic nature of these symptoms adds an emotional layer of distress, affecting mood and overall well-being.

The protracted nature of RA can also contribute to psychological challenges, with anxiety and depression being prevalent companions for those navigating the intricacies of the condition. Furthermore, the visible joint deformities and physical changes wrought by RA may exert an influence on body image and self-esteem, demanding individuals to navigate a complex psychological landscape.

In response to these challenges, individuals with RA frequently employ an array of adaptations and coping mechanisms. Lifestyle modifications become imperative, prompting adjustments in home environments, integrating adaptive tools, and adopting assistive devices to preserve independence. Effective coping strategies are crucial for managing the emotional toll, encompassing mindfulness practices, stress-reduction techniques, and seeking support from mental health professionals and support groups.

The impact of RA on relationships is a dynamic facet that necessitates nuanced consideration. Family dynamics may undergo shifts as roles and responsibilities are recalibrated to accommodate the needs of the individual with RA. Intimate relationships can be influenced by physical limitations and the emotional impact of the condition, underscoring the significance of open communication and mutual understanding.

In navigating the intricacies of Rheumatoid Arthritis, a comprehensive approach that addresses not only the physical symptoms but also the emotional, psychological, and social dimensions is imperative. Tailored interventions, spanning medical management, emotional support, and adaptive strategies, constitute the bedrock for enhancing the overall well-being of those affected by RA and mitigating its impact on their quality of life.

Chapter Two: The Diagnosis Journey

Embarking on the diagnostic journey of Rheumatoid Arthritis (RA) encompasses critical facets without section numbers. This chapter guides you through the diagnostic process, unraveling the significance of standard tests employed. Effective communication with healthcare providers becomes paramount, emphasizing the pivotal role of advocating for oneself.

Delving into the emotional impact of an RA diagnosis, coping strategies are offered to foster acceptance. Furthermore, friends, family, and support groups play an instrumental role in building a robust support system, nurturing open communication within this pivotal network that aids in navigating the complexities of the diagnostic path.

The Diagnostic Process

Embarking on the diagnostic journey for Rheumatoid Arthritis (RA) involves a systematic process comprising distinct steps and crucial tests to decipher the complexities of this autoimmune disorder.

Clinical Assessment

Clinical assessment is the bedrock of the diagnostic process for Rheumatoid Arthritis (RA), serving as an intricate examination of the patient's symptoms and physical presentation. Patient history, the initial facet of this process, holds significant weight as it unveils essential contextual information. Inquiring about joint symptoms' duration, intensity, and progression establishes a temporal framework and sheds light on potential triggers. This historical context lays the foundation for a more nuanced understanding of the patient's journey with RA.

Symptom examination, the next crucial step, involves a meticulous review of persistent joint pain, swelling, and stiffness. This examination not only identifies affected joints but also assesses their impact on daily life. Tenderness, warmth, and the presence of deformities contribute to a refined diagnostic picture, enabling healthcare providers to tailor interventions to the specific needs of the individual.

Functional assessment delves into the practical implications of RA symptoms on daily activities. This evaluation gauges the severity of the condition by assessing the patient's ability to perform routine tasks. The findings here provide valuable insights into the disease's impact on the patient's quality of life, guiding an adequate treatment plan formulation.

Joint examination, a hands-on exploration of joints, is pivotal for assessing tenderness, swelling, and range of motion. Identifying specific joint involvement is crucial for tailoring a targeted diagnostic and treatment approach. Extra-articular manifestations, such as nodules or systemic symptoms like fatigue, are also considered, providing a comprehensive view of RA beyond its impact on joints.

Patient-reported outcomes, encompassing pain intensity, fatigue levels, and overall well-being, offer a subjective perspective. This information, directly from the patient, adds a layer of understanding to the clinical assessment, reflecting the individual's experience of RA. Integrating patient-reported outcomes into the diagnostic process ensures a more holistic and patient-centered approach to care.

Finally, the psychosocial assessment, considering emotional well-being and the broader impact of RA on mental health, completes the clinical evaluation. This component recognizes that RA affects the body and the individual's overall well-being. Understanding these psychosocial aspects is crucial for tailoring comprehensive care and support strategies that address the holistic needs of individuals navigating the complexities of Rheumatoid Arthritis.

Blood Test

Blood tests constitute a critical dimension in the diagnostic toolkit for Rheumatoid Arthritis (RA), offering intricate insights into the autoimmune and inflammatory processes associated with this complex condition. Each blood test serves a specific role, contributing to a nuanced understanding of the disease's manifestation.

Rheumatoid Factor (RF): Rheumatoid factor, an antibody that targets healthy tissues, is a critical marker in RA diagnostics. Elevated RF levels in blood suggest an autoimmune response. While not exclusive to RA, a positive RF test prompts further investigation into the autoimmune nature of the condition.

Anti-Citrullinated Protein Antibodies (ACPAs): ACPAs, antibodies targeting citrullinated proteins prevalent in RA, provide a definite indicator. Their presence in blood strongly suggests RA and aids in differentiating it from other arthritic conditions. A positive ACPA test is instrumental in confirming RA diagnosis.

C-Reactive Protein (CRP) and Erythrocyte Sedimentation Rate (ESR): CRP and ESR serve as markers of systemic inflammation. Elevated levels in the blood indicate heightened inflammatory activity. While not exclusive to RA, these markers contribute valuable information about the overall inflammatory burden and guide the assessment of disease activity.

Complete Blood Count (CBC): CBC comprehensively analyzes blood components, including red and white blood cells. Anemia, a common occurrence in RA due to chronic inflammation, can be identified through CBC. An elevated white blood cell count may indicate active inflammatory processes.

Liver and Kidney Function Tests: Monitoring liver and kidney function is crucial in RA management, considering the impact of certain medications on these organs. Regular tests ensure the safe use of medications, and abnormal results prompt adjustments in treatment plans, emphasizing the importance of a holistic approach to care.

Anti-Nuclear Antibodies (ANA): Although not specific to RA, the presence of ANAs in blood may indicate autoimmune activity. Positive ANA results necessitate further investigations to discern the underlying cause, contributing to a comprehensive understanding of the autoimmune landscape.

Appreciating the intricacies of each blood test empowers healthcare providers to construct a detailed diagnostic profile. The convergence of positive RF and ACPA tests, complemented by elevated CRP and ESR levels, establishes a robust foundation for RA diagnosis. These tests confirm the autoimmune nature of the disease and guide healthcare providers in formulating precise and individualized treatment strategies for those navigating the complexities of Rheumatoid Arthritis.

Imaging Studies

Imaging studies constitute a crucial dimension in the diagnostic armamentarium for Rheumatoid Arthritis (RA), offering detailed insights into joint health and aiding in the nuanced assessment of disease progression. Each imaging modality contributes distinct perspectives, enriching the comprehensive understanding of RA's impact on the musculoskeletal system.

X-Rays: X-rays serve as the foundational imaging tool, offering a static yet invaluable assessment of joint health. They detect characteristic features of RA, including joint damage, erosions, and potential deformities. Over time, X-rays provide a longitudinal view, capturing changes in affected joints and contributing essential information about structural alterations indicative of RA.

Magnetic Resonance Imaging (MRI): MRI, a sophisticated imaging modality, provides detailed views of bone and soft tissues. In RA, MRI becomes a crucial tool for assessing inflammation, identifying early joint damage, and comprehensively understanding disease activity. This modality excels in revealing the subtleties of RA's impact on joint structures, aiding in the formulation of targeted and precise treatment strategies.

Ultrasound: Ultrasound emerges as a dynamic imaging tool, offering real-time visualization of joints. Its effectiveness lies in detecting synovitis, a hallmark of RA, and assessing joint effusions. Ultrasound's real-time capabilities allow for a dynamic evaluation, providing insights into the inflammatory processes within joints and guiding interventions based on immediate observations.

Dual-Energy X-ray Absorptiometry (DEXA): DEXA scans extend beyond joint assessment to evaluate bone mineral density. Given the increased risk of osteoporosis in individuals with RA, DEXA scans become instrumental in the early detection of bone density changes. This proactive approach facilitates timely interventions to mitigate the risk of fractures, addressing a crucial aspect of RA-related complications.

Computed Tomography (CT) Scans: While less commonly employed in routine RA diagnostics, CT scans offer detailed cross-sectional images of joints and surrounding structures. In specific cases where detailed imaging is imperative, such as assessing bony erosions or complications, CT scans may provide valuable information complementing other imaging modalities.

Appreciating the nuanced roles of each imaging modality empowers healthcare providers to tailor their diagnostic approach to the specific needs of individuals with RA. X-rays lay the groundwork for structural assessment, while advanced modalities like MRI and ultrasound offer dynamic insights into inflammation and early damage. Integrating imaging studies into the diagnostic process enhances the precision of RA assessments, facilitating informed decision-making in the comprehensive management of Rheumatoid Arthritis.

Synovial Fluid Analysis

Synovial fluid analysis is a pivotal diagnostic tool in assessing Rheumatoid Arthritis (RA), providing crucial insights into the inflammatory processes occurring within affected joints. This procedure involves the aseptic aspiration of synovial fluid from the affected joint, typically performed with a thin needle. The collected synovial fluid undergoes microscopic examination to assess its cellular composition, with an elevated white blood cell count, particularly an abundance of neutrophils, indicating active inflammation.

Biochemical analysis of synovial fluid includes evaluating levels of proteins, enzymes, and other substances. Elevated levels of inflammatory markers, such as C-reactive protein (CRP) and erythrocyte sedimentation rate (ESR), corroborate the presence of inflammation. Additionally, assessing glucose levels helps rule out infectious causes.

Identifying crystals, such as urate or calcium pyrophosphate crystals, in synovial fluid aids in differentiating RA from other arthritic conditions. This contributes to a precise and tailored approach to treatment, ensuring that individuals receive interventions targeted to their specific condition.

Synovial fluid analysis serves as a direct indicator of active inflammation within the joint, aiding in the accurate assessment of disease activity. The insights gained from this analysis play a crucial role in guiding treatment decisions and formulating a personalized and effective treatment plan for managing RA. Serial synovial fluid analyses over time provide a longitudinal perspective on disease progression, assisting healthcare providers in evaluating the effectiveness of treatment interventions and making timely adjustments as needed.

In summary, synovial fluid analysis, with its detailed examination of cellular and biochemical components, stands as a cornerstone in the diagnostic arsenal for RA. By providing a direct window into the inflammatory processes within the joint, this procedure informs accurate diagnosis, guides treatment strategies, and facilitates ongoing monitoring of Rheumatoid Arthritis.

Diagnostic Criteria

Diagnostic criteria in Rheumatoid Arthritis (RA) are standardized guidelines healthcare providers use to establish a definitive diagnosis, providing a systematic approach to identifying individuals with the disease.

One notable set of criteria is the 1987 American College of Rheumatology (ACR) criteria, supplemented by the 2010 ACR/European League Against Rheumatism (EULAR) criteria. These criteria incorporate a combination of clinical and laboratory findings, including the presence and duration of joint symptoms, serological markers such as rheumatoid factor and anti-citrullinated protein antibodies, acute phase reactants, and joint involvement.

The significance of these diagnostic criteria lies in their multifaceted contributions to the diagnostic process. Firstly, they facilitate early identification of RA, enabling healthcare providers to initiate timely interventions. Early diagnosis is paramount for effective disease management, preventing irreversible joint damage, and improving long-term outcomes for individuals with RA.

Secondly, the diagnostic criteria ensure precision in diagnosis by considering a range of disease manifestations. By incorporating clinical symptoms, serological markers, and imaging findings, these criteria minimize the risk of misdiagnosis and contribute to accurately identifying RA. This precision is essential for tailoring appropriate treatment strategies based on the specific disease characteristics of each individual.

Moreover, the diagnostic criteria guide healthcare providers in making informed treatment decisions. Once RA is accurately diagnosed, these criteria help determine the most suitable interventions, including the initiation of disease-modifying antirheumatic drugs (DMARDs) or other targeted therapies. This tailored approach to treatment improves disease management and enhances the overall quality of care.

The significance of diagnostic criteria also extends to the standardization of assessment. By providing a structured framework for diagnosis, these criteria promote consistency in identifying RA among healthcare providers and across different clinical settings. This standardization ensures that individuals with RA receive a uniform and comprehensive evaluation, regardless of the healthcare setting.

Lastly, the dynamic nature of diagnostic criteria is crucial. As our understanding of RA advances, diagnostic criteria evolve to incorporate new knowledge. This ongoing refinement ensures that the criteria remain aligned with the latest insights into the disease, reflecting the dynamic nature of RA research and enhancing diagnostic accuracy.

In conclusion, diagnostic criteria in Rheumatoid Arthritis are essential tools that contribute significantly to the diagnostic process. Their multifaceted significance lies in enabling early identification, ensuring precision in diagnosis, guiding treatment decisions, promoting standardized assessment, and evolving with the latest advancements in our understanding of RA.

Meticulously considering each step in the diagnostic process is imperative for accurate RA diagnosis. This comprehensive approach empowers healthcare providers to tailor interventions, initiate timely treatments, and collaboratively navigate the complexities of

Rheumatoid Arthritis with the individual, optimizing overall health outcomes.

Communicating with Healthcare Providers

Effectively communicating with healthcare providers regarding Rheumatoid Arthritis (RA) is a nuanced and crucial aspect of managing this chronic condition. This goes beyond the surface-level exchange of symptoms; it involves active advocacy, holistic dialogue, and a continuous commitment to shared decision-making throughout the diagnostic journey and ongoing care.

Clear and open communication forms the bedrock for an accurate diagnosis and the development of targeted treatment plans for RA. As key contributors to their healthcare, individuals play a pivotal role in conveying the intricacies of their symptoms—detailing the nature, duration, and intensity. This transparency serves as the basis upon which healthcare providers build a comprehensive understanding of the disease's impact on an individual's life.

Moreover, effective communication extends to the development of personalized treatment plans. An open discourse encompassing symptoms, treatment preferences, and lifestyle factors empowers individuals to engage in decision-making actively. This collaborative approach ensures that treatment strategies align not only with clinical necessities but also with the unique needs and preferences of the individual, fostering a sense of ownership over their healthcare journey.

Regular and transparent communication remains essential for monitoring disease activity and treatment efficacy. Updates on changes in symptoms, potential side effects, and overall well-being provide healthcare providers with real-time insights, allowing for timely adjustments to the treatment plan. This proactive engagement enhances the precision of disease management, contributing to improved long-term outcomes.

Rheumatoid Arthritis is not solely a physical challenge; it significantly impacts an individual's emotional well-being. Effective communication provides a platform for individuals to express the emotional challenges associated with RA, such as stress, anxiety, or the psychological toll of chronic pain. This holistic dialogue enables healthcare providers to offer tailored support, including mental health resources and coping strategies, fostering comprehensive well-being.

Advocacy is paramount, particularly during the diagnostic journey. Individuals are encouraged to be proactive advocates for their health by providing a detailed medical history. This includes not only the specifics of RA symptoms but also familial autoimmune conditions and relevant past health issues. This comprehensive information empowers healthcare providers to navigate the diagnostic process more effectively.

Self-advocacy extends to expressing concerns, preferences, and treatment goals. A proactive stance ensures that healthcare decisions align with an individual's values and lifestyle, fostering a collaborative and patient-centered approach. Seeking clarification on medical information and treatment options is integral to this advocacy, ensuring individuals have a nuanced understanding of their condition and the proposed interventions.

Active participation in shared decision-making is a cornerstone of effective communication. This collaborative process involves a partnership between individuals and healthcare providers, ensuring that treatment decisions are informed by clinical expertise and the individual's unique experiences. Actively engaging in shared decision-making fosters a sense of empowerment and mutual understanding, contributing to treatment plans that are more likely to be adhered to and successful.

Ensuring regular follow-up and consistent communication is vital. This ongoing dialogue facilitates the tracking of progress, the assessment of treatment outcomes, and the prompt addressing of emerging concerns. The dynamic nature of RA demands a responsive and patient-centered approach to care, which is only possible through sustained and open communication.

In conclusion, effective communication in the context of Rheumatoid Arthritis is a multifaceted and ongoing dialogue that encompasses advocacy, holistic consideration of emotional well-being, and active participation in shared decision-making. By fostering this nuanced and collaborative approach, individuals with RA can contribute to a healthcare journey that is clinically effective and tailored to their unique needs, ultimately leading to improved disease management and overall well-being.

Coping with a New Diagnosis

Coping with a new diagnosis of Rheumatoid Arthritis (RA) is a profound and often challenging experience that encompasses emotional impacts and the development of coping strategies for acceptance and well-being.

The emotional impact of receiving an RA diagnosis can be overwhelming. Individuals may face various emotions, including shock, fear, anger, and grief. The realization of living with a chronic condition that can affect daily life and overall well-being may evoke a sense of uncertainty about the future. Furthermore, the potential adjustments to daily routines, concerns about pain and mobility, and the perceived loss of control over one's body can contribute to heightened emotional distress.

Navigating these emotions is an integral part of the coping process. Emotional well-being is closely tied to the overall management of

RA, and acknowledging and addressing these feelings is crucial for holistic care. Healthcare providers play a pivotal role in supporting individuals through this emotional journey, offering resources such as counseling, support groups, and educational materials to help individuals understand and manage the emotional impact of their diagnosis.

Developing strategies for coping and acceptance is essential for adapting to life with RA. These strategies can encompass a variety of aspects:

Education and Understanding: Knowledge is empowering. Learning about RA, its treatment options, and potential lifestyle adjustments can help individuals feel more in control and better equipped to manage the condition.

Building a Support System: Creating a strong support network is crucial. This includes friends, family, and fellow individuals with RA who can provide understanding, empathy, and practical assistance. Support groups, either in person or online, can offer a sense of community and shared experiences.

Mind-Body Techniques: Practices such as mindfulness, meditation, and deep breathing exercises can help manage stress and anxiety associated with the diagnosis. These techniques promote a sense of calm and contribute to overall emotional well-being.

Adapting Daily Routines: Making practical adjustments to daily routines and activities can help individuals maintain a sense of normalcy. This may involve finding alternative ways to perform tasks, incorporating regular breaks, and prioritizing self-care activities.

Setting Realistic Goals: Establishing realistic and achievable short-term and long-term goals fosters a sense of accomplishment and control. Celebrating small victories and progress, no matter how incremental, contributes to a positive mindset.

Engaging in Physical Activity: Exercise tailored to individual capabilities can be crucial in managing RA symptoms. It not only contributes to physical well-being but also releases endorphins, which can positively impact mood.

Open Communication: Discussing concerns and feelings with healthcare providers, friends, and family fosters open communication. This transparency allows for a collaborative approach to managing RA and ensures that support is available when needed.

Accepting the diagnosis is a continuous process, and individuals may find that their coping strategies evolve over time. It's essential to recognize that emotional responses to a new RA diagnosis are valid and that seeking support and employing coping mechanisms contribute to a more resilient and positive outlook on living with the condition. The journey of coping and acceptance is unique to each individual. With time, many find a way to integrate RA into their lives while maintaining a fulfilling and meaningful existence.

Building a Support System

Establishing a robust support system is a pivotal and intricate process, particularly when confronted with the life-altering diagnosis of Rheumatoid Arthritis (RA). The support system, comprising friends, family, and participation in support groups, becomes an intricate web of emotional sustenance, practical assistance, and open communication, addressing the multifaceted challenges associated with RA.

Friends and Family

Friends and family, functioning as emotional pillars during the diagnostic phase, extend beyond providing a mere support structure. Their roles become profound as individuals grapple with the emotional impact of the RA diagnosis. Beyond the physical toll, RA can evoke a spectrum of emotions—shock, fear, anger, and grief. Loved ones provide a crucial foundation for coping with these emotions by offering unwavering support, empathy, and a nuanced understanding.

Practical assistance from friends and family becomes indispensable as RA often necessitates significant adjustments in daily life. From aiding with household tasks to providing transportation and companionship during medical appointments, their tangible support alleviates the physical strain associated with RA.

Moreover, loved ones play a crucial role in educating themselves about RA. This knowledge transforms them into effective advocates within the familial setting and broader social circles. Their understanding fosters an environment of empathy and awareness, contributing to a more supportive and informed network.

Participation in Support Groups

Participation in support groups offers an additional layer of understanding and connection. These groups become invaluable spaces where individuals share similar experiences, challenges, and triumphs. The benefits include shared experiences that create a sense of camaraderie, practical advice for managing symptoms drawn from real-world experiences, and emotional validation.

Beyond emotional connection, support groups provide a wealth of practical advice. Members share strategies for managing symptoms, navigating the healthcare system, and adapting to lifestyle changes. This collective wisdom empowers individuals with insights from real-world experiences, fostering a more informed and proactive approach to managing RA.

Being part of a support group provides a platform for emotional expression without fear of judgment. The shared journey of RA fosters emotional validation, affirming that the myriad feelings associated with the diagnosis are not only understandable but shared by others in the community.

Encouraging Open Communication

Encouraging open communication within the support network is crucial for fostering understanding and creating an environment of empathy. Individuals need to feel at ease expressing their needs, whether for physical assistance, emotional support, or specific accommodations. This transparent communication cultivates a supportive environment where everyone is on the same page, fostering a more holistic and collaborative approach to managing RA.

Moreover, support groups and open communication channels contribute to a more dynamic and interconnected support system. This interconnectedness becomes an invaluable resource as individuals navigate the complexities of living with RA. Friends, family, and support groups collectively create a resilient network that empowers individuals to confront the challenges of RA with a sense of community and understanding, ultimately contributing to a more nuanced and practical approach to managing the condition.

Chapter Three: Medical Management and Treatment

In exploring Medical Management and Treatment for Rheumatoid Arthritis (RA), this chapter provides a comprehensive overview of diverse treatment options, underscoring the crucial need for personalized plans. It emphasizes their integral role in RA management by delving into common medications and therapeutic approaches.

The discussion extends to lifestyle modifications, incorporating insights on integrating diet, exercise, and sleep into the treatment plan. Furthermore, the chapter stresses the imperative of seeking professional help, emphasizing building a collaborative relationship with healthcare professionals for nuanced and tailored care fostering a holistic and patient-centered approach to RA management.

Overview of Treatment Options

The effective management of Rheumatoid Arthritis (RA) necessitates a nuanced understanding of various treatment options, each playing a distinctive role in addressing the complexity of this autoimmune condition. The introduction to these treatment approaches encompasses a spectrum of interventions, including medications, therapeutic modalities, and lifestyle modifications.

Medications may range from nonsteroidal anti-inflammatory drugs (NSAIDs) and disease-modifying antirheumatic drugs (DMARDs) to biologics, each serving specific purposes in symptom control, inflammation reduction, and disease progression mitigation. Therapeutic approaches often involve physical and occupational therapies, aiming to enhance joint function and manage daily activities amidst RA-related challenges.

Concurrently, lifestyle modifications, such as dietary adjustments, regular exercise, and sleep hygiene, contribute significantly to overall RA management. Central to this comprehensive landscape is the imperative of crafting a personalized treatment plan. Recognizing that RA manifests uniquely in each individual, a tailored approach is indispensable.

Customizing treatment plans considers factors such as age, overall health, specific RA symptoms, comorbidities, and lifestyle. This individualized strategy optimizes interventions' effectiveness and acknowledges each patient's diverse needs and circumstances.

The importance of a personalized treatment plan extends beyond mere symptom management. It encompasses the broader aspects of an individual's life, addressing emotional well-being, daily routines, and long-term goals. Involving patients in decision-making empowers them, fostering a sense of ownership and commitment to their treatment journey. The collaboration between healthcare providers and patients in developing a personalized plan is pivotal, as it not only tailors interventions to the specific needs of the individual but also enhances treatment adherence and overall therapeutic outcomes.

Medication and Therapies

Managing Rheumatoid Arthritis (RA) involves a multifaceted approach, encompassing an exploration of common medications and therapeutic strategies and a nuanced understanding of their pivotal role in navigating the complexities of this chronic autoimmune condition.

Exploration of Common Medications

Nonsteroidal Anti-Inflammatory Drugs (NSAIDs)

Nonsteroidal Anti-Inflammatory Drugs (NSAIDs) represent a crucial component in the arsenal of medications used to manage Rheumatoid Arthritis (RA). This class of medications encompasses a range of drugs, including well-known examples such as Ibuprofen and Naproxen. The role of NSAIDs in RA management is multifaceted, focusing primarily on providing symptomatic relief from pain and inflammation associated with the disease.

NSAIDs exert their therapeutic effects by inhibiting the activity of enzymes called cyclooxygenases (COX). These enzymes are pivotal in producing prostaglandins, contributing to inflammation, pain, and fever. By blocking COX, NSAIDs reduce the production of prostaglandins, leading to a decrease in inflammatory processes and alleviation of associated symptoms.

One of the primary roles of NSAIDs in RA management is to provide immediate relief during acute flare-ups. RA is characterized by periods of increased disease activity, marked by intensified joint inflammation and pain. NSAIDs act swiftly to mitigate these symptoms, offering patients a reprieve from the discomfort associated with heightened disease activity.

While NSAIDs are effective for short-term symptomatic relief, their long-term use requires careful consideration. Prolonged and indiscriminate use of NSAIDs may be associated with potential side effects, particularly concerning the gastrointestinal (GI) and cardiovascular systems. Gastrointestinal complications, such as ulcers and bleeding, are known risks associated with NSAID use. Additionally, specific NSAIDs may pose an increased risk of cardiovascular events.

The effectiveness of NSAIDs can vary among individuals, and healthcare providers often need to tailor the choice of NSAID based on factors such as the patient's overall health, medical history, and the presence of other conditions. Some individuals may respond better to one NSAID over another, emphasizing the importance of personalized treatment plans.

NSAIDs are frequently incorporated into a comprehensive treatment plan for RA, which may include other medications such as disease-modifying antirheumatic drugs (DMARDs) or corticosteroids. Coordinated care ensures that each component of the treatment plan complements the others, providing optimal relief while minimizing potential side effects.

Patients using NSAIDs for RA management require regular monitoring by healthcare professionals to assess their response to treatment and watch for any signs of adverse effects. Patient education is a crucial aspect of NSAID use, involving discussions about proper dosages, potential side effects, and the importance of reporting any unusual symptoms promptly.

In conclusion, NSAIDs play a vital role in the management of RA by providing rapid symptomatic relief during flare-ups. Their use, however, necessitates a thoughtful and individualized approach, considering both the immediate needs of the patient and potential long-term implications. When integrated into a well-coordinated treatment plan and accompanied by regular monitoring and patient education, NSAIDs contribute significantly to enhancing the quality of life for individuals living with Rheumatoid Arthritis.

Disease-Modifying Antirheumatic Drugs (DMARDs)

Disease-Modifying Antirheumatic Drugs (DMARDs) constitute a pivotal class of medications in the holistic approach to managing Rheumatoid Arthritis (RA). This diverse group of drugs plays a crucial role in not only alleviating symptoms but also modifying the course of the disease, aiming to slow or halt its progression and prevent irreversible joint damage.

Conventional DMARDs, such as Methotrexate and Hydroxychloroquine, form the backbone of RA treatment. Methotrexate, inhibiting folate metabolism, is often the initial choice, effectively slowing disease progression and preserving joint function. Consistent monitoring is essential to address potential side effects effectively. Hydroxychloroquine, with its immunomodulatory properties, is particularly useful in mild to moderate RA and is often prescribed in combination with other DMARDs. Regular eye examinations are essential due to ocular toxicity risk during long-term use.

Biologic DMARDs offer a more targeted approach. Tumor Necrosis Factor (TNF) Inhibitors, including Etanercept, Adalimumab, and Infliximab, target TNF, a key inflammatory cytokine, reducing inflammation and preventing joint damage. They are deployed when conventional DMARDs are insufficient, with regular infection monitoring. Non-TNF Biologics, like Rituximab and Abatacept, act on different immune system components and are considered in cases where TNF inhibitors are ineffective or not tolerated. Infusion reactions and infections require vigilant monitoring, and administration often occurs in a healthcare setting.

The role of DMARDs in RA management is pivotal, aiming to suppress the overactive immune response responsible for joint inflammation and damage. These medications play a crucial role in achieving sustained disease control, preserving joint function, and improving the overall quality of life for individuals with RA.

Personalized treatment plans are paramount in DMARD therapy. Healthcare providers tailor these plans based on individual factors such as disease severity, comorbidities, and patient preferences. This personalized approach ensures the optimal balance between effectiveness and safety for each patient.

In some instances, a combination of DMARDs, both conventional and biologic, may be prescribed to enhance therapeutic efficacy. Combination therapy is especially considered when a single DMARD is insufficient in controlling RA symptoms.

Regular monitoring is essential for individuals on DMARD therapy due to the potential for side effects. This includes routine assessments for laboratory parameters, imaging studies, and vigilant observation for any signs of adverse effects. Regular communication between patients and healthcare providers ensures timely adjustments to the treatment plan.

In conclusion, DMARDs, encompassing both conventional and biologic forms, stand as cornerstones in the comprehensive management of Rheumatoid Arthritis. Their disease-modifying properties, when integrated into personalized and monitored treatment plans, contribute significantly to the well-being of individuals navigating the complexities of RA.

Corticosteroids

Corticosteroids, a class of potent anti-inflammatory medications, are pivotal in addressing the complex landscape of Rheumatoid Arthritis (RA). Operating distinctively from anabolic steroids, corticosteroids wield significant influence in alleviating inflammation and mitigating the symptomatic challenges associated with RA.

Corticosteroids exert their therapeutic effects by modulating the immune response and curbing inflammation. Acting at the cellular level, they influence gene expression and inhibit the production of pro-inflammatory substances. Available in various forms, including oral tablets, injectable solutions, topical creams, and intra-articular injections, corticosteroids offer flexibility in administration tailored to the severity and specific requirements of RA treatment.

Oral corticosteroids find utility for short-term relief during acute symptoms or as a temporary bridge during disease flares. However, prolonged use is generally avoided due to the risk of systemic side effects, including bone density loss, weight gain, increased blood pressure, and heightened susceptibility to infections.

Intra-articular injections directly into affected joints are a common approach for localized relief, providing targeted anti-inflammatory effects. Careful management of the frequency of these injections is essential to prevent potential joint damage, with healthcare providers considering the overall treatment plan when incorporating this form of corticosteroid therapy.

Topical corticosteroids, applied as creams or ointments to the skin over affected joints, offer localized relief from symptoms, proving particularly useful for managing skin involvement in RA, such as rheumatoid nodules.

While corticosteroids are effective in symptom management, they have potential side effects. These can include mood changes, insomnia, elevated blood sugar levels, and, with prolonged use, more severe complications like osteoporosis and adrenal gland suppression.

Corticosteroids often play a role as part of a comprehensive RA treatment plan, providing rapid relief from inflammation during disease flares. However, their long-term use is carefully weighed against potential side effects, and efforts are made to minimize reliance on corticosteroids to maintain overall health.

In the context of patient-centric care, the use of corticosteroids is highly individualized. Healthcare providers consider factors such as the patient's overall health, specific RA manifestations, and the presence of comorbidities when incorporating corticosteroids into the treatment regimen.

In conclusion, corticosteroids emerge as versatile tools in managing RA, offering rapid relief from inflammation and symptoms. Their judicious use within the broader treatment context underscores the delicate balance between therapeutic benefits and potential side effects, aiming to optimize the overall quality of care for individuals navigating the complexities of Rheumatoid Arthritis.

Exploration of Therapeutic Approaches

Physical Therapy

In Rheumatoid Arthritis (RA) management, physical therapy assumes a multifaceted role aimed at optimizing joint health and overall mobility. Customized exercises are designed to enhance joint function, improve muscle strength, and maintain mobility.

The nuanced approach of physical therapists considers the specific needs of individuals, tailoring programs that not only alleviate symptoms but also contribute to sustained physical well-being.

Incorporating progressive exercises, range-of-motion activities, and targeted interventions reflects a commitment to fostering long-term joint health and improving the overall quality of life for those grappling with RA.

Occupational Therapy

Occupational therapy stands as a cornerstone in the comprehensive care of individuals with RA, focusing on the practical aspects of daily living. This therapeutic avenue adapts activities to accommodate joint limitations and integrates assistive devices for optimized functionality. Beyond physical adaptation, the role of occupational therapy extends to enhancing independence and equipping individuals with effective coping strategies.

By addressing the unique challenges presented by RA in the context of daily activities, occupational therapy becomes an empowering force, enabling individuals to navigate their routines with increased ease, confidence, and a sense of control.

Complementary Therapies

In the diverse landscape of RA management, complementary therapies offer an array of supplementary approaches that extend beyond conventional medical interventions. Examples such as acupuncture, massage, and hydrotherapy provide additional avenues for pain relief and contribute to overall physical and mental well-being. These therapies are often integrated into treatment plans alongside standard medical approaches, creating a holistic and personalized strategy. Considerations for incorporating complementary therapies revolve around their role in enhancing the effectiveness of conventional treatments, fostering a balanced and comprehensive approach to RA management that acknowledges the multidimensional nature of the condition.

In the dynamic interplay of physical therapy, occupational therapy, and complementary therapies, individuals with RA are presented with a nuanced and tailored approach to their care. This comprehensive strategy not only addresses the immediate symptoms of the condition but also recognizes and supports the broader dimensions of well-being, fostering a sense of empowerment and active participation in the journey towards improved health.

The exploration of common medications and therapeutic approaches, coupled with a profound understanding of their roles in RA management, forms the cornerstone of a holistic and effective strategy for individuals navigating the challenges of Rheumatoid Arthritis. This comprehensive approach, guided by ongoing collaboration between patients and healthcare providers, ensures a tailored and responsive care plan that addresses immediate symptoms and long-term disease management.

Lifestyle Modifications

A fundamental aspect of navigating Rheumatoid Arthritis (RA) lies in integrating lifestyle modifications as indispensable components of a holistic management strategy. The collaborative journey between individuals and healthcare providers involves in-depth discussions to tailor these adjustments to the unique needs and challenges posed by RA.

Dietary considerations assume a nuanced role, transcending a mere focus on nutrition. The emphasis lies in cultivating an anti-inflammatory dietary framework encompassing diverse nutrient-rich foods. This includes a spectrum of fruits, vegetables, whole grains, and lean proteins strategically infused with omega-3 fatty acids, recognized for their anti-inflammatory properties. The collaborative efforts with healthcare providers ensure the alignment of dietary choices with the specific goals of RA management and a broader perspective that acknowledges individual nutritional requirements.

Physical activity emerges as a dynamic and personalized facet of lifestyle modifications, extending beyond the conventional understanding of exercise. Tailored exercise programs, meticulously curated in consultation with physical therapists, are designed to go beyond symptom alleviation. They prioritize activities that not only enhance joint function but also contribute to improved muscle strength and overall fitness. The deliberate integration of regular exercise into daily routines fosters a proactive and sustainable approach to maintaining joint health.

The spotlight on lifestyle modifications extends to the realm of sleep hygiene, recognizing the profound impact of restorative sleep on overall well-being. Establishing consistent sleep routines, optimizing sleep environments, and managing factors such as pain or discomfort become integral components. Adequate and restful sleep complements the body's natural healing processes and amplifies the effectiveness of other therapeutic interventions.

In this comprehensive approach, lifestyle modifications transcend mere routine adjustments; they become empowering tools for individuals with RA. This holistic strategy complements medical interventions and fosters a profound sense of agency and resilience by addressing the intricate interplay of diet, physical activity, and sleep. It encapsulates a nuanced understanding of living with Rheumatoid Arthritis, acknowledging the multifaceted challenges and providing a personalized roadmap for navigating the complexities of this autoimmune condition.

Seeking Professional Help

Central to the effective management of Rheumatoid Arthritis (RA) is the proactive engagement with healthcare professionals, underscoring the importance of seeking tailored care and fostering a collaborative relationship with the healthcare team.

A fundamental tenet of RA management involves stressing the paramount importance of consulting healthcare professionals. This emphasis is rooted in recognizing that RA is a complex and variable condition, necessitating specialized expertise for optimal care. As key healthcare team members, rheumatologists play a central role in diagnosis, treatment planning, and ongoing monitoring.

Collaboration with other specialists, such as physical, occupational, and nutritionists, contributes to a comprehensive and multidisciplinary approach. Beyond the expertise offered by specialists, regular check-ups and ongoing communication with healthcare professionals become integral components of tailored care.

Monitoring disease activity, assessing treatment efficacy, and addressing emerging concerns are vital aspects of this collaborative journey. Individuals with RA are encouraged to actively participate in these consultations actively, providing valuable insights into their experiences and preferences, ultimately contributing to the customization of their care plan.

Collaborative care extends beyond mere consultation to establishing a true partnership between individuals and their healthcare teams. This collaboration is characterized by open communication, mutual respect, and shared decision-making. Individuals' proactive and engaged stance empowers them to articulate their goals, express concerns, and actively participate in decisions regarding their treatment plans.

The collaborative relationship involves addressing the immediate medical needs and considering the broader aspects of well-being. Healthcare professionals work collaboratively to integrate lifestyle modifications, mental health support, and strategies for coping with the emotional challenges associated with RA into the overall care plan.

Central to this collaboration is the recognition that the management of RA is a dynamic and evolving process. Regular follow-ups, ongoing adjustments to the treatment plan, and a responsive approach to changing needs contribute to developing a care strategy that aligns with the individual's unique journey with RA.

In essence, seeking professional help in RA management transcends the conventional patient-provider dynamic. It embodies a collaborative partnership where healthcare professionals' expertise converges with individuals' lived experiences and preferences, forging a path toward tailored and comprehensive care. This approach not only addresses the complexities of RA but also empowers individuals to actively navigate the challenges of living with this autoimmune condition.

Chapter Four: Navigating Daily Life with RA

Within the scope of living with Rheumatoid Arthritis (RA), the chapter on Navigating Daily Life serves as a comprehensive guide to managing the multifaceted challenges of this condition. It unveils Workplace Strategies, addressing the intricacies of professional life while managing RA, fostering effective communication, and offering solutions for workplace challenges.

Delving into Social Relationships and RA, it navigates maintaining connections amidst the condition's impact on relationships. Moreover, Traveling with RA receives attention with valuable tips for symptom management during travels. Additionally, Self-Care Practices highlight the vital role of personalized routines in RA management, enriching this chapter as a compass for daily life with RA.

Workplace Strategies

Navigating the professional landscape while managing Rheumatoid Arthritis (RA) requires a comprehensive and strategic approach, considering the challenges inherent to the condition and the nuances of effective communication in a workplace setting. Managing RA in the workplace involves a nuanced understanding of potential hurdles individuals may encounter. These challenges encompass a spectrum, ranging from physical limitations affecting daily tasks to the necessity for flexible work arrangements to accommodate the variable nature of RA symptoms.

Addressing these challenges necessitates implementing practical solutions to create an inclusive and supportive work environment. For instance, ergonomic adjustments to the workspace, such as specialized chairs or adaptive tools, can significantly alleviate strain on joints, promoting a more comfortable and sustainable work routine.

Flexibility in work hours or the option for remote work stands as a critical solution, accommodating fluctuations in symptoms and promoting a healthier work-life balance. Collaborating with employers to establish a workplace culture that prioritizes support and inclusivity is essential for successfully implementing these solutions.

Transparent and effective communication emerges as a cornerstone in developing workplace strategies for RA. While the decision to disclose the RA diagnosis remains personal, communicating specific needs with employers becomes crucial. This may involve discussing the need for ergonomic adjustments, occasional flexibility in work hours, or other accommodations that enhance overall work productivity. Regular check-ins with employers to discuss workloads, deadlines, and potential adjustments foster a proactive and supportive work dynamic, ensuring that the work environment remains attuned to the needs of individuals managing RA.

Communication extends beyond employers to colleagues, and effective interactions are pivotal in cultivating a supportive work culture. Educating colleagues about RA, its impact, and potential adjustments fosters empathy and understanding. Open communication about specific needs ensures that colleagues are aware and equipped to offer support when necessary. Creating a mutual support and understanding culture enhances the overall work experience for individuals managing RA, contributing to a positive and inclusive workplace environment.

In essence, workplace strategies for managing RA go beyond addressing challenges; they encompass creating an accommodating and actively supportive workplace culture. By implementing practical solutions and fostering transparent communication with employers and colleagues, these strategies aim to empower individuals with RA to thrive in their professional pursuits while effectively managing the conditions' complexities.

Social Relationships and RA

The impact of Rheumatoid Arthritis (RA) extends beyond the physical realm, influencing various aspects of an individual's life, including social relationships. Navigating the intricacies of maintaining and fostering social connections while addressing challenges posed by RA requires a delicate balance and proactive strategies.

Maintaining a robust social life is integral to overall well-being, and individuals with RA often find solace, support, and joy in their social connections. Nurturing relationships with friends, family, and the broader community can provide emotional support, encouragement, and a sense of normalcy amid the challenges posed by RA.

Engaging in social activities, whether in-person or virtually, allows individuals with RA to stay connected with their support network, fostering a sense of belonging and mitigating the potential isolation that can accompany chronic health conditions. RA can introduce unique relationship challenges, requiring open communication and mutual understanding.

Physical limitations, unpredictable symptom flare-ups, and the emotional toll of managing a chronic condition can impact various facets of relationships. Individuals with RA and their loved ones must engage in honest and compassionate conversations about the condition's implications. This includes discussing the potential adjustments needed in daily activities, acknowledging the emotional impact of RA, and establishing a supportive environment.

In intimate relationships, partners may need to adapt to changes in physical intimacy or provide additional assistance during periods of increased symptom severity. Open communication about the challenges and adjustments required fosters a collaborative approach to navigating the impact of RA on the relationship. Partners, family members, and friends can play a vital role in offering emotional support, understanding the fluctuating nature of RA symptoms, and actively managing the condition.

In the broader social sphere, individuals with RA may encounter misconceptions or lack of awareness about their condition. Advocating for oneself, educating friends and acquaintances about RA, and setting boundaries when necessary contribute to fostering understanding and supportive social interactions. Social support groups, both online and in-person, can also provide a valuable space for individuals with RA to connect with others who share similar experiences, offering empathy, shared coping strategies, and a sense of community.

In essence, navigating social relationships with RA involves a dynamic interplay of maintaining connections, fostering understanding, and addressing challenges collaboratively. By embracing open communication, advocating for one's needs, and actively participating in social activities, individuals with RA can cultivate a supportive network that enhances their overall well-being and resilience in the face of the unique challenges posed by the condition.

Traveling with RA

For individuals with Rheumatoid Arthritis (RA), embarking on a journey requires a meticulous and comprehensive strategy to navigate the unique challenges posed by the condition. Beyond the typical considerations of travel planning, managing RA during trips involves a thoughtful approach to symptom management, ensuring a seamless and enjoyable travel experience. Let's delve into a detailed exploration of strategies tailored to the practical and emotional aspects of traveling with RA.

Tips for Managing RA Symptoms While Traveling

Packing Essentials: In addition to the standard travel essentials, individuals with RA should curate a specialized packing list. This includes prescribed medications, joint support aids such as braces or wraps, and thermal packs for quick relief during flare-ups. A compact first aid kit containing over-the-counter pain relievers and necessary prescription medications adds an extra layer of preparedness.

Planning Regular Breaks: Acknowledging the potential worsening of joint stiffness during prolonged periods of immobility, meticulous trip planning should incorporate regular breaks. These intervals allow for stretching, movement, and changes in position, mitigating stiffness and contributing to overall comfort and well-being.

Hydration and Nutrition: Recognizing the impact of dehydration on joint discomfort, individuals with RA should prioritize staying hydrated and maintaining a balanced diet. Carrying a refillable water bottle and nourishing snacks is essential. Considering dietary preferences or restrictions during travel planning ensures that meals align with individual needs.

Adapting Seating Arrangements: Thoughtful consideration of seating arrangements is crucial, regardless of the mode of transportation. Individuals with RA should explore additional legroom and supportive seating options, whether on a plane, train, or car. Carrying unique cushions or pillows tailored to specific needs enhances comfort during extended periods of sitting.

Managing Medications Effectively: Consistency in medication management is paramount. Travelers should carry medications in their original packaging, accompanied by a written list of prescriptions. Maintaining a record of medication schedules ensures adherence, especially when navigating different time zones or adjusting to changes in daily routines.

Preparing for Trips and Ensuring a Smooth Travel

Choosing Accommodations Wisely: Delving into the details of accommodations is essential. Selecting lodgings with accessibility features, such as elevators, ramps, and comfortable bedding, contributes significantly to a pleasant stay. Proactively communicating with the chosen lodging about specific needs ensures necessary preparations are in place.

Informing Travel Companions: Transparent communication with travel companions about RA and its potential impact is a cornerstone of a successful trip. Open discussions about specific needs and potential adjustments in plans and fostering an understanding of the condition create a supportive and collaborative travel environment.

Securing Travel Insurance: Acknowledging the unpredictable nature of chronic conditions, individuals with RA should consider securing comprehensive travel insurance. This coverage offers financial protection in the face of unexpected medical expenses, providing peace of mind throughout the journey.

Researching Medical Facilities at the Destination: Acquiring knowledge about the location of medical facilities at the destination is a prudent preparatory step. Identifying nearby hospitals, clinics, and pharmacies ensures quick access to medical assistance if needed, contributing to a more confident and relaxed travel experience.

Utilizing Assistive Devices: Tailoring travel plans to include assistive devices, such as walking aids, wheelchairs, or mobility scooters, significantly enhances independence and accessibility. Planning ahead to ensure the availability of these devices at the destination ensures a smooth and accommodating travel experience.

In essence, traveling with RA demands a meticulous and proactive approach that addresses the journey's practical and emotional dimensions. By integrating these detailed strategies, individuals with RA can manage their symptoms effectively during travel and enhance the overall experience. The journey becomes an opportunity for enrichment, resilience, and the celebration of the indomitable spirit that defines those navigating life with Rheumatoid Arthritis.

Self-Care Practices

In the intricate tapestry of managing Rheumatoid Arthritis (RA), the pivotal role of self-care emerges as a guiding thread, weaving together the physical, emotional, and mental aspects of well-being. Far beyond a mere luxury, self-care becomes a fundamental strategy for individuals navigating the nuanced landscape of RA symptoms. This comprehensive exploration delves into the multifaceted layers of self-care, elucidating its profound significance and offering a nuanced perspective on crafting a personalized routine tailored to the unique needs of those living with RA.

Significance of Self-Care in RA Management

The journey of living with RA is often marked by the daily negotiation of chronic pain, joint stiffness, and the unpredictable nature of symptom flare-ups. In this complex terrain, self-care transcends a mere set of practices; it becomes a proactive and empowering strategy to enhance overall health and mitigate the specific challenges posed by RA. The merits of integrating self-care into the daily routine of individuals with RA are manifold.

Firstly, self-care serves as a potent tool for pain management. Through gentle exercises, heat therapies, and mindful practices, individuals can navigate and alleviate the persistent discomfort associated with RA. Stress reduction is another crucial facet of self-care. Given the interplay between stress and RA symptoms, engaging in relaxation techniques such as meditation and deep breathing exercises becomes pivotal in fostering a sense of calm and resilience.

Furthermore, self-care contributes to enhanced mobility, mitigating the impact of RA on daily activities. Tailored exercises, including joint-friendly activities like swimming or yoga, play a pivotal role in maintaining flexibility and strength without exacerbating joint strain. Emotionally, self-care becomes a sanctuary for individuals navigating the emotional toll of RA. Creative outlets, such as art or writing, provide an expressive medium to process emotions, fostering emotional well-being.

Crafting a Personalized Self-Care Routine

The art of self-care is inherently personal, necessitating a bespoke approach that aligns with individual needs and preferences. A personalized self-care routine encompasses a spectrum of activities designed to cater to the unique challenges and aspirations of individuals with RA.

Physical exercise assumes a central role in this customized routine. Gentle yet effective activities, such as swimming or tai chi, contribute to maintaining joint flexibility and strength and serve as therapeutic outlets. Mindfulness and relaxation techniques, ranging from meditation to guided imagery, offer individuals the tools to manage stress and anxiety effectively.

Applying heat and cold therapies is a cornerstone in the self-care toolkit, providing targeted relief from pain and inflammation. Dietary considerations become integral; incorporating anti-inflammatory foods into daily meals supports overall health and complements the management of RA symptoms. Prioritizing adequate and quality sleep is non-negotiable, with a consistent bedtime routine and a sleep-friendly environment contributing to optimal sleep hygiene.

Engaging in creative pursuits, such as painting or gardening, fosters emotional well-being and provides an outlet for self-expression. Social connection is not overlooked; nurturing relationships and participating in activities with loved ones contribute to a sense of community and emotional support.

In summary, the journey of self-care in RA management extends far beyond routine practices. It is a holistic and dynamic endeavor, acknowledging the intricate interplay of physical and emotional well-being. By embracing self-care principles and tailoring them to individual preferences, individuals with RA can forge a path toward resilience, effective symptom management, and an enriched quality of life.

Chapter Five: Coping with Flare-ups

Within the unpredictable journey of Rheumatoid Arthritis (RA), flare-ups stand as tempests, challenging the equilibrium carefully maintained by individuals. This chapter delves into the nuanced art of navigating these storms, offering insights into identifying triggers, deploying coping strategies, adjusting daily activities, and maintaining crucial communication with healthcare providers.

Understanding common triggers becomes paramount, as does developing personalized coping mechanisms for managing pain and emotional distress during flare-ups. Balancing daily activities by modifying routines and seeking timely guidance from healthcare providers completes the toolkit for confronting and weathering RA flare-ups.

Identifying Triggers

In the complex landscape of Rheumatoid Arthritis (RA), the experience of flare-ups introduces a multifaceted challenge, demanding a comprehensive understanding of the triggers that can disrupt the delicate equilibrium individuals strive to maintain. This in-depth exploration seeks to navigate the intricate realm of identifying triggers, encompassing widely recognized factors contributing to RA flare-ups and personalized strategies for discerning individual sensitivities.

RA flare-ups can be triggered by a diverse range of factors, constituting a foundational aspect of proactive management. Stress, a pervasive contributor, exerts a profound impact on RA symptoms, often amplifying inflammation and precipitating flare-ups. Weather changes, specifically variations in humidity and temperature, emerge as influential factors affecting joint pain and stiffness in individuals with RA.

Engaging in physical exertion or strenuous activities without adequate pacing is a potential trigger, emphasizing the need for thoughtful activity management. Moreover, certain foods, particularly those known for their inflammatory properties, can contribute significantly to RA symptoms, necessitating a closer examination of dietary habits.

The recognition that triggers vary considerably from individual to individual underscores the importance of adopting a personalized and meticulous approach to trigger identification. Strategies for discerning personal triggers include maintaining a comprehensive symptom journal. This involves systematically documenting daily activities, emotional states, and dietary intake to provide an invaluable reference for discerning patterns and potential triggers.

Environmental observations play a crucial role, with individuals paying close attention to changes in weather conditions and potential exposure to allergens to identify external contributors to flare-ups. Stress management techniques, such as meditation, yoga, or mindfulness, not only aid in identifying emotional triggers but also serve as proactive measures to mitigate their impact. Dietary exploration takes the form of a systematic assessment of the impact of different foods on symptoms through a structured process of elimination and reintroduction, allowing for pinpointing potential dietary triggers.

By amalgamating a thorough understanding of general triggers with a personalized exploration of individual sensitivities, individuals with RA empower themselves to anticipate and manage flare-ups more effectively. This proactive and tailored approach enhances the overall quality of life and establishes a foundation for informed and constructive dialogues with healthcare providers. The result is a collaborative and holistic approach to RA management that acknowledges the uniqueness of each individual's journey.

Coping Strategies During Flare-ups

Rheumatoid Arthritis (RA) flare-ups introduce a multifaceted set of challenges, demanding an intricate and holistic strategy to address the intricate interplay of physical and emotional dimensions. In this detailed exploration, we unfold an extensive toolkit of coping strategies, offering profound insights into managing the multifaceted aspects of pain and discomfort while cultivating resilience in the face of emotional strain.

Practical Tips for Managing Pain and Discomfort

Mindful Movement: Incorporating gentle, low-impact exercises, such as tailored stretching routines or yoga sequences, into daily life is a foundational pillar for managing pain. These activities not only enhance flexibility but also provide relief from joint stiffness without exacerbating existing pain, contributing holistically to overall well-being.

Heat and Cold Therapy: The dynamic strategy of alternating between heat and cold applications offers a nuanced approach to pain relief. Warm compresses strategically applied to stiff joints provide soothing comfort, while cold packs effectively reduce inflammation, addressing discomfort and the underlying inflammatory processes.

Medication Adherence: A critical aspect of managing flare-ups lies in strict adherence to prescribed medications. The judicious use of anti-inflammatory drugs and pain relievers, guided by healthcare providers, plays a pivotal role in mitigating symptoms. Open communication with healthcare professionals ensures a personalized medication regimen tailored to individual needs.

Joint Protection Techniques: Implementing joint protection strategies is imperative to minimize discomfort and enhance quality of life. This includes the judicious use of assistive devices, such as braces or splints, and thoughtful modification of daily activities to reduce strain on affected joints, offering practical adjustments that contribute significantly to pain management.

Emotional Coping Mechanisms

Mindfulness and Relaxation Techniques: Cultivating mindfulness through practices like deep breathing, progressive muscle relaxation, or guided imagery provides a sanctuary for emotional well-being. These techniques foster relaxation and equip individuals to manage the emotional toll of flare-ups, promoting a holistic approach to symptom management.

Social Support: Establishing and maintaining connections with friends, family, or support groups becomes a vital emotional resource during flare-ups. Shared experiences and empathetic understanding within a supportive network help alleviate the sense of isolation that can accompany flare-ups. Open communication about emotional challenges fosters a sense of community and shared strength.

Creative Outlets: Engaging in creative pursuits through art, writing, or music offers a therapeutic channel for expressing emotions. Creative expression serves as a cathartic release, diverting focus from pain and providing a meaningful outlet for self-expression, contributing to emotional well-being.

Professional Support: Recognizing the impact of emotional challenges seeking the guidance of a mental health professional becomes a valuable component of coping during flare-ups. Tailored strategies and therapeutic interventions offer individuals a proactive approach to managing emotional well-being, fostering resilience and a sense of empowerment.

Navigating RA flare-ups demands a delicate balance between managing physical symptoms and nurturing emotional resilience. By integrating a spectrum of practical pain management techniques with effective emotional coping mechanisms, individuals with RA can not only weather the storm of flare-ups but also emerge with a profound sense of empowerment and a fortified capacity to navigate the challenges of living with RA.

Adjusting Daily Activities

Rheumatoid Arthritis (RA) flare-ups present a unique challenge, necessitating a thoughtful adjustment of daily activities to manage the impact on physical well-being. This detailed exploration unveils a comprehensive approach, offering insights into the nuanced process of modifying routines during flare-ups while striking a delicate balance between activity and rest.

In modifying daily routines, prioritizing tasks based on urgency and physical demand becomes essential. During flare-ups, identifying key activities and allocating energy effectively ensures that crucial responsibilities are addressed without exacerbating discomfort. Efficient time management practices are paramount, including breaking tasks into smaller, manageable segments with scheduled rest intervals to distribute physical exertion evenly throughout the day, minimizing strain on affected joints.

Additionally, incorporating assistive devices, such as ergonomic tools or adaptive equipment, aids in simplifying daily activities, reducing the strain on joints and enabling individuals to engage in tasks with greater ease during flare-ups. Balancing activity and rest is a delicate art requiring a keen understanding of one's body signals.

Attuning oneself to the body's signals becomes crucial, recognizing early signs of fatigue or discomfort to allow for proactive adjustments and promoting a balanced approach that prevents overexertion. Integrating intentional rest periods into the daily schedule is vital, offering regular breaks, even for short durations, to provide the body with opportunities to recuperate and minimize the cumulative impact of physical activity.

Ensuring quality sleep is an integral aspect of balancing activity and rest, involving creating a conducive sleep environment, adhering to a consistent sleep schedule, and practicing relaxation techniques that contribute to overall well-being during flare-ups. Strategic planning plays a key role, involving the spacing out of energy-intensive activities and the incorporation of adequate rest intervals, preventing the build-up of fatigue and optimizing the utilization of available energy throughout the day.

Adapting work environments to accommodate ergonomic principles is crucial for individuals navigating flare-ups. Modifying workspaces with proper chair height, keyboard positioning, and desk layout minimizes strain on joints, contributing to a more comfortable and supportive work environment. Exploring flexible work arrangements, such as telecommuting or adjusting work hours when feasible, supports individuals in adapting their professional responsibilities to the challenges posed by flare-ups.

Incorporating leisure activities into the daily routine requires mindful choices that align with physical capabilities during flare-ups. Opting for low-impact exercises, gentle hobbies, or activities that promote relaxation fosters enjoyment without exacerbating symptoms. Engaging in adaptive strategies for leisure, such as exploring seated versions of activities or incorporating assistive devices, ensures that individuals can continue to participate in fulfilling and enjoyable pursuits during flare-ups.

Navigating daily life during RA flare-ups involves a delicate dance of modification and rest. By adopting a thoughtful approach to daily routines, individuals can strike a balance that promotes well-being, minimizes discomfort, and allows for the continued pursuit of meaningful activities despite the challenges posed by flare-ups.

Communicating with Healthcare Providers During Flares

Navigating Rheumatoid Arthritis (RA) flare-ups necessitates a proactive and collaborative relationship with healthcare professionals, emphasizing the significance of timely communication and the need for adjustments to treatment plans. This comprehensive exploration delves into the crucial role of communication in managing flares, highlighting the importance of open dialogue between individuals with RA and their healthcare team.

Importance of Timely Communication

Monitoring Symptom Changes: Timely communication begins with a vigilant awareness of changes in RA symptoms. Individuals are encouraged to monitor fluctuations in pain, stiffness, swelling closely, and overall joint function during flare-ups, providing a foundation for effective communication with healthcare providers.

Recognizing Early Warning Signs: The ability to recognize early warning signs of a flare is paramount. Educating individuals about potential indicators, such as increased fatigue, changes in sleep patterns, or heightened inflammation markers, empowers them to initiate communication with healthcare providers at the onset of flare-related challenges.

Preventing Escalation of Symptoms: Timely communication serves as a proactive measure to prevent the escalation of symptoms. By promptly addressing changes in RA activity, healthcare providers can collaboratively intervene, potentially minimizing the duration and severity of flares through timely adjustments to treatment plans.

Seeking Guidance and Adjustments to Treatment

Collaborative Treatment Plans: A collaborative approach to treatment involves open discussions between individuals and their healthcare team. Seeking guidance during flare-ups initiates a dialogue about the current symptomatology, enabling healthcare providers to tailor interventions based on the specific needs and challenges presented by the individual.

Adjusting Medications: Flare-ups often necessitate adjustments to medication regimens. Timely communication allows healthcare providers to evaluate the effectiveness of current medications, explore potential modifications, or introduce additional therapies to address the heightened inflammatory activity characteristic of flares.

Addressing Emotional Well-being: Effective communication extends beyond physical symptoms to encompass emotional well-being. Sharing the emotional impact of flare-ups with healthcare providers facilitates a holistic understanding of the individual's experience, enabling the incorporation of psychosocial support into the overall treatment plan.

Providing Feedback on Treatment Efficacy: Individuals are encouraged to actively participate in discussions about the efficacy of current treatments during flare-ups. Sharing insights into how treatments impact daily life, including side effects or challenges, enables healthcare providers to fine-tune interventions for optimal results.

Empowering Individuals in Their RA Journey

Encouraging Advocacy: Timely communication empowers individuals to advocate for their needs. Encouraging a proactive approach to sharing information about flare-related challenges fosters a sense of agency, positioning individuals as active participants in their RA management.

Building a Trusting Relationship: Establishing and nurturing a trusting relationship with healthcare providers is foundational to effective communication. Open dialogue, built on mutual trust and respect, creates an environment where individuals feel comfortable discussing the nuances of their RA experience, enhancing the quality of care provided.

Facilitating Informed Decision-Making: Informed decision-making is facilitated through transparent communication. Individuals armed with comprehensive information about their RA, treatment options, and potential adjustments are better equipped to engage actively in decisions that impact their health and well-being.

Navigating RA flare-ups is dynamic, and effective communication forms the bedrock of successful management. By recognizing the importance of timely communication, seeking guidance during flares, and actively participating in treatment discussions, individuals with RA can forge a collaborative alliance with their healthcare providers, enhancing the precision and efficacy of their overall management strategy.

Chapter Six: Looking Towards the Future

As we venture into the concluding chapter, we focus on the future landscape of Rheumatoid Arthritis (RA) management. This section intricately examines the long-term outlook for RA, shedding light on both the prognosis and the exciting strides in research and forthcoming treatment options.

Beyond the medical spectrum, the chapter probes into the often-overlooked domain of financial considerations, providing insights into the economic impact of RA and equipping readers with resources to navigate healthcare costs. Advocacy and empowerment are underscored, urging readers to engage within the healthcare system proactively. The chapter concludes with a glimpse into ongoing research and emerging treatments, hinting at potential breakthroughs that hold promise for the future of RA care.

Long-Term Outlook for RA

The long-term outlook for Rheumatoid Arthritis (RA) is multifaceted, influenced by various elements that define an individual's journey with this chronic autoimmune condition. Prognosis relies heavily on early detection, timely commencement of appropriate treatment, and the unique response of each patient to therapeutic measures. Early diagnosis often translates to improved outcomes, including effective symptom management, preservation of joint function, and an enhanced quality of life. Customizing treatment plans to suit individual needs is crucial, emphasizing the significance of a collaborative approach between patients and healthcare providers, significantly shaping a more favorable prognosis.

The landscape of RA management is undergoing a remarkable transformation, driven by ongoing advancements in research and the emergence of promising treatment avenues. Scientific breakthroughs unraveling the molecular intricacies and genetic aspects of RA have led to the development of targeted therapies and innovative biologic medications. These therapeutic interventions aim to alleviate symptoms and modify the course of the disease, representing a comprehensive evolution in RA treatment.

Biologics, disease-modifying anti-rheumatic drugs (DMARDs), and targeted therapies signify progress in tailoring treatments to suit individual characteristics, offering more effective and well-tolerated options. The horizon of RA management continues to expand with emerging research areas such as gene therapies and advanced biologics, holding the potential to further refine treatment approaches and enhance outcomes for individuals with RA.

The interplay between personalized care and groundbreaking treatments underscores a transformative future in RA management. This evolving landscape holds promise, not just in symptom control but in the potential modification of the underlying disease processes. The synergy between patient-centered care and cutting-edge research signifies a future where RA management is more effective and intricately attuned to the unique needs and experiences of each person navigating Rheumatoid Arthritis.

As our understanding of RA deepens and research progresses, the trajectory for individuals grappling with this condition becomes increasingly optimistic. Collaborative patient-provider relationships and the integration of personalized care pave the way for a more hopeful outlook. The evolving treatment paradigms in RA management herald a future where improved outcomes and a more patient-centric approach redefine the journey for individuals with Rheumatoid Arthritis.

Financial Considerations

Living with Rheumatoid Arthritis (RA) extends beyond the physical and emotional challenges, as it also involves navigating the complex financial implications associated with managing a chronic condition. The financial impact of RA can be substantial, encompassing not only direct medical expenses but also indirect costs that may arise from adjustments to work life and daily living due to the condition's effects. As individuals with RA grapple with these financial considerations, adopting a thoughtful and strategic approach becomes imperative.

The financial implications of RA are multifaceted, often posing challenges for individuals and their families. Direct medical expenses include the costs associated with regular doctor visits, laboratory tests, imaging studies, and the ongoing need for medications. The cumulative effect of these expenses can create a significant economic burden, particularly for those without comprehensive health insurance coverage.

Moreover, individuals with RA may face indirect costs related to productivity loss at work, potential disability, and the need for additional support services, further amplifying the economic challenges. Fortunately, various resources are available to help individuals cope with the financial challenges of RA. Government programs, non-profit organizations, and pharmaceutical assistance programs may offer financial support or access to discounted medications.

Exploring these resources is essential for individuals seeking relief from the economic strain of managing a chronic condition, ensuring that necessary medical care remains accessible. Strategies for managing healthcare costs within the context of RA involve proactive communication with healthcare providers. Engaging in open discussions about treatment options, potential generic alternatives, and considerations for financial constraints can lead to collaborative decision-making that aligns with medical needs and financial realities. Additionally, exploring options for prescription assistance programs, generic medications, or therapeutic alternatives can contribute to more cost-effective healthcare without compromising the quality of treatment.

For those navigating the financial landscape of RA, proactive financial planning becomes a crucial aspect of overall well-being. This includes understanding insurance coverage, exploring available assistance programs, and developing a comprehensive budget for medical and daily living expenses. Seeking guidance from financial counselors or support groups can provide valuable insights and personalized strategies for managing the economic aspects of living with RA.

In conclusion, addressing the financial considerations associated with RA is integral to comprehensive care for individuals with this condition. By understanding the multifaceted financial impact, exploring available resources, and implementing effective strategies, individuals with RA can better navigate the economic challenges while prioritizing their health and overall well-being.

Advocacy and Empowerment

In managing Rheumatoid Arthritis (RA), advocacy and empowerment emerge as powerful tools, allowing individuals to shape their journey with this chronic condition actively. Advocacy involves raising awareness about RA and encouraging individuals to assert their needs within the healthcare system. Conversely, empowerment entails fostering a proactive mindset, enabling individuals to take charge of their RA journey with confidence and resilience.

Encouraging readers to advocate for themselves within the healthcare system is paramount for optimal RA management. This advocacy starts with effective communication with healthcare providers. Individuals with RA are encouraged to openly discuss their symptoms, treatment preferences, and any challenges faced in adhering to the prescribed treatment plan. Through assertive communication, individuals can ensure that their unique needs and concerns are acknowledged, leading to more tailored and effective care.

Furthermore, advocating for oneself in the healthcare system involves staying informed about RA, treatment options, and emerging therapies. Proactively seeking information empowers individuals to participate in decision-making about their treatment journey. This might include understanding the potential side effects of medications, exploring alternative therapies, and staying abreast of advancements in RA research. A well-informed advocate is better equipped to collaborate with healthcare providers, providing a more personalized and effective treatment plan.

Empowering individuals to be proactive in their RA journey is integral to fostering a sense of control and resilience. Proactivity extends beyond medical appointments and treatment decisions; it involves actively managing one's overall well-being. This may include adopting a healthy lifestyle through regular exercise, maintaining a balanced diet, and prioritizing adequate sleep. Proactive self-care measures contribute to improved physical and emotional resilience, positively impacting the overall RA experience.

Empowerment in the context of RA also means cultivating a support network. Building connections with others facing similar challenges, joining support groups, and participating in advocacy initiatives create a sense of community. This shared experience fosters a supportive environment where individuals can exchange insights, strategies, and encouragement, reinforcing the belief that they are not alone in their journey.

In conclusion, advocacy and empowerment are pivotal to navigating life with Rheumatoid Arthritis. Encouraging individuals to advocate for themselves within the healthcare system and empowering them to be proactive in their RA journey contributes to a more personalized and resilient approach to managing this chronic condition. By embracing these principles, individuals with RA can shape a path that aligns with their unique needs, preferences, and aspirations.

Research and Emerging Treatments

The ever-evolving landscape of Rheumatoid Arthritis (RA) management is illuminated by the beacon of ongoing research, which explores innovative treatments and potential breakthroughs. This continuous journey into the realm of scientific inquiry not only deepens our understanding of RA and holds the promise of transformative advancements that can reshape the narrative of those living with this chronic condition.

The current state of research in RA is characterized by a diverse array of investigations encompassing genomics, immunology, and cutting-edge imaging technologies. Researchers are unraveling the intricate mechanisms underpinning RA, seeking to demystify its complexity and identify novel therapeutic targets. This multidimensional approach contributes to developing more targeted and personalized treatment strategies that address the unique characteristics of RA in individual patients.

A closer look at ongoing research unveils a dynamic interplay between fundamental science discoveries and their translation into clinical applications. Genomic studies not only shed light on the genetic factors influencing RA susceptibility but also pave the way for precision medicine approaches that tailor treatments based on an individual's genetic profile. Immunological investigations delve into the intricacies of the immune response, uncovering potential points of intervention to modulate disease activity.

Biologic therapies, a hallmark of recent advancements, have revolutionized RA treatment by explicitly targeting immune system components involved in the disease process. As ongoing research refines our understanding of these biologics, the horizon expands to include novel agents and optimized treatment strategies. Small molecules, offering an oral alternative to injectable biologics, add another layer of diversity to the treatment landscape, catering to individual preferences and needs.

Exploring emerging treatments extends beyond the traditional boundaries, embracing regenerative medicine approaches. Stem cell therapies and tissue engineering potentially revolutionize RA management by promoting joint repair and modulating the immune response at its root. These regenerative strategies represent a frontier where science and medicine collaborate to offer transformative solutions.

The collaboration between researchers, pharmaceutical companies, and healthcare providers is critical to the progression of research.

Clinical trials, as pivotal conduits for translating scientific discoveries into tangible treatment options, provide individuals with RA the opportunity to access cutting-edge therapies while contributing to the collective knowledge that propels the field forward.

However, as we anticipate breakthroughs in RA treatment, it is paramount to approach emerging therapies with a balanced perspective. Rigorous evaluation of safety, efficacy, and long-term outcomes is essential to ensure that the promises of these treatments translate into meaningful benefits without compromising overall well-being.

In conclusion, the journey of research and emerging treatments in Rheumatoid Arthritis offers a tapestry of possibilities. Staying informed about the latest advancements empowers individuals and healthcare providers and fosters a sense of optimism for a future where RA management is more nuanced, personalized, and effective. As the horizon of possibilities unfolds, the scientific community and individuals' collective effort shapes a future where RA becomes a condition that can be navigated with greater precision and hope.

Conclusion

As we conclude this in-depth exploration into navigating life with Rheumatoid Arthritis (RA), reflecting on the rich tapestry of insights woven throughout these pages is paramount. Our journey has been a comprehensive expedition, unraveling the intricate layers of RA, from its defining characteristics to the nuanced strategies for medical management and holistic treatment. Beyond the clinical aspects, we've delved into the lived experiences and challenges individuals with RA encounter daily.

In revisiting the wealth of information, our primary objective has been to empower readers with a profound understanding of RA. This understanding guides individuals to make informed decisions tailored to their unique circumstances. From the crucial aspects of early diagnosis and symptom recognition to the exploration of diverse management strategies, our discussions have aimed to equip readers with the knowledge needed to navigate the complexities of RA with confidence and resilience.

As we step away from the detailed discussions, it is crucial to underscore the fundamental messages that echo throughout this guide. The significance of early diagnosis, the collaborative relationship with healthcare professionals, and the individualized nature of RA management are not just information but guiding principles for those traversing the unpredictable terrain of RA.

Peering into the future, the path may be veiled in uncertainties, yet within these uncertainties lies the strength and resilience of individuals living with RA. The journey is a testament to the daily courage, adaptability in the face of challenges, and the unwavering spirit that propels each step forward. To every person facing the trials of RA, know that your journey is unique yet shared in the collective experience of a community that understands and supports.

In conclusion, let us acknowledge and celebrate the resilience of those living with RA. The road may twist and turn, but with each twist comes an opportunity for growth, discovery, and triumph. The challenges of RA do not define your journey but the strength with which you navigate them. As you move forward, may your path be illuminated by moments of joy, a robust support network, and the unshakable belief in your ability to navigate life with Rheumatoid Arthritis. The pages of this guide may close, but the story of resilience, hope, and strength unfolds in the chapters yet to be written.

Dear Valued Reader,

We trust that the exploration of "Navigating Rheumatoid Arthritis" has provided you with knowledge and support. Your engagement with this guide is immensely valuable, and we would be honored to hear your reflections. If the content has resonated with you, we invite you to share your thoughts on platforms such as Amazon, Goodreads, or any other review site you prefer.

Your review not only aids us in refining our work but also serves as a beacon for others navigating similar journeys with Rheumatoid Arthritis. Your honest feedback is integral to our collective effort to provide understanding, resilience, and guidance within the RA community.

We genuinely appreciate the time and consideration you invest in sharing your thoughts. Your reviews transcend words; they become pillars of support for those seeking empowerment on their journey with Rheumatoid Arthritis. Thank you for being an indispensable part of this shared commitment.

With heartfelt thanks and warm regards,

Edna Walton,

Author of Navigating Rheumatoid Arthritis.

www.ingramcontent.com/pod-product-compliance
Lightning Source LLC
Chambersburg PA
CBHW060952260726
48661CB00005B/1861